Miserable Joy

Chronic Pain in the Christian Life

Jason M. Nelson

From Heartache To Healing

Northwestern Publishing House
Milwaukee, Wisconsin

Third printing, 2014
Second printing, 2009

Cover photos: ShutterStock, Inc.
Art Director: Karen Knutson
Designer: Pamela Dunn

Library of Congress Control Number: 2005925578
Northwestern Publishing House
1250 N. 113th St., Milwaukee, WI 53226-3284
www.nph.net

Published 2007
Printed in the United States of America
ISBN 978-0-8100-1749-8

To my beautiful, steady wife, Nancy,
who has willingly suffered many things with me.

To Amanda, Laura, Justin, and Jordan who knew when it was
the pain talking and gave their father the benefit of the doubt.

To my granddaughters, Abigail and Noelle, whose precious smiles
always remind me that as long as there is life, there is hope.

Contents

Introduction

Only in the mind of God could suffering and joy coexist. A paradox of such monumental proportions would never have occurred to us. That is because his thoughts are so above our thoughts and his ways beyond figuring out. Only by the grace of God can we have pain and be happy at the same time. That can only be true because Jesus was tested in every way that we are—and accomplished for us what we could never have accomplished for ourselves—and has promised to be with us always, everywhere, and through everything. The life and work of Jesus interplay with everything that happens to Christians. That is what living by faith is all about. The Lord's fingerprint is on everything in our lives. Sometimes he permits Satan, or circumstances, to alter the lives of his people, and then God cleans up spotlessly afterward. But at the end of the day, or a lifetime, what God ordains is always good. So when relentless pain works God's purpose in our lives, it resolves in many ways, including joy. Sometimes a very *miserable joy.*

God never intended for the creatures he created to suffer. He loves us; he loves his whole creation. In the beginning it was all very good. Pain and paradise are mutually exclusive. Pain wasn't on his radar at the dawn of time, at least not as we know it now. But it was in his toolbox. And when human disobedience threatened to undermine his cosmic plan, it didn't take him long to reach for the pain tool and make it an inevitable and productive part of the human experience. As a result, we now experience pain in childbirth, pain-wracked illnesses, work that can be filled with pain, emotions that can be crippled with pain. At the same time, the pain we experience can also instruct, shape, and develop us like nothing else can. Only of the mind of God could it be said, "Consider it pure joy, my brothers, whenever you face trials of many kinds, because you know that the testing of your faith develops perseverance. Perseverance must finish its work so that you may be mature and complete, not lacking anything" (James 1:2-4).

Let's be real. No one celebrates the onset of pain, hoping it will last long enough to hammer new character traits out of a recalcitrant and sinful life. No psychologically healthy person asks God to bring on pain or tries to inflict it on himself. But when pain comes and stays, God is at work. Absolutely nothing is outside of his promise that in *all things* he works for good for those who love him. Not the pain of loneliness, migraines, cancer, clinical depression, mental illness, MS, broken relationships, or a badly wrecked back. We pray for God to take the pain away. We pray for miraculous healing. But when pain is our constant companion, we also bargain with God to take the pain away, promising to be better the next time around. And then, as the pain hangs on and won't let go, we realize this is not a little life lesson from God. This is a life redesigned for purposes that exist first and only in the mind of God—the reorganization of a life to accomplish his holy will. This too is a gift of God's grace in Christ, and it will work for good.

This is not a book about pain in any medical sense. It is not a book about pain management techniques. It is not a book filled with pretense or platitudes that don't square with someone else's personal reality. And it is absolutely not intended to be a book about me. It is a book about living. It is a book about the rigorous exercise of faith—mind, body, and spirit—that is required to live a Christian life while battling chronic pain. Writing this book was not easy for a lot of reasons, but it was a necessary way for me to express the miserable joy of my life with chronic pain.

Experience is a powerful teacher. Our experiences help us mature. Painful as some of our experiences can be, they can also inspire new thoughts and understandings within us and help us develop new competencies. For better or worse, we cannot escape the impact of our experiences.

Dear friend, if pain is the experience God has given you, use it.

Chapter 1

The **Pain** of Pain

Pain is a very subjective phenomenon. While everyone has experienced pain, no two people have experienced it the same way. What might be irritating to one pain sufferer could be debilitating for someone else. People in pain have a lot in common, but no one really knows what another person is going through. Only God knows what each of us is going through because he is there in it.

My pain story is the classic, worst-case, back pain scenario. Your pain story might be something entirely different. I pray that you can relate to some of the things I share with you. I pray that you will be able to see yourself on these pages and find something helpful and encouraging as you battle your pain. I also pray that you will reflect on the love of God that is very much at work in your life, and the purposes which God might still be making known to you.

Until I became a pain person, I had a very narrow definition of *pain.* Now I know that pain is complex and layered. It has physiological, psychological, emotional, and spiritual dimensions. I have learned that defining and describing pain is very important while working with doctors and other pain specialists. *It hurts* just doesn't cut it like it used to. Now I have to decide if my pain is burning, throbbing, aching, deep, superficial, radiating, or tingling. I have to give it a rating of 1 to 10 under a range of different circumstances. I have to draw where it is located on the backside and front side of naked male forms that remind me I will soon be stripped of any modesty I brought with me to the pain clinic. More pain on pain. The exercise of defining and describing my pain causes me a fair amount of anxiety before each visit. I mentally rehearse what I want to say and how I want to say it. I want to be accurate. And yet I am worried about saying too much or too little. I really don't like talking about my pain.

Maybe that is because pain rarely stands alone in the human experience. Often it is accompanied by many other issues, which the pain sufferer has to work through.

The first definition of *pain* in my little Merriam-Webster's dictionary is most unfortunate: "1. punishment, penalty." Then comes, "2. suffering or distress of body or mind." What a terrible burden that first definition places on the heart of a Christian suffering pain!

The Bible is clear: when sin entered the world through human rebellion, the consequences were horrible. The ill and harm we suffer in this life are clearly the result of being sinful people and living in a sin-filled world. But it would be devastating to faith and life to conclude that chronic personal pain is some kind of special punishment from God for something he just doesn't like about that individual. Nothing could be more false. God more than likes us; he loves us in an amazing-grace kind of way. He inflicted the worst possible pain on himself through the suffering and death of his Son, Jesus. He did it because he, himself, *is* love. His mercy will trump anything else that is going on in our lives. Through faith in Jesus, we live in grace and not in fear of punishment. The apostle Paul made this very distinction when he wrote that there is no condemnation of any kind for those who are in Christ Jesus (Romans 8:1). Pain may be the consequence of a lot of things that we bring on ourselves. Pain may be the hard evidence that God is shaping and molding us to be different than we were. But please read this right: *Pain is not punishment.* Don't let the worst pain of pain become guilt.

The topic of pain management is on the lively edge in the medical community. Pain clinics are springing up across the country and becoming major divisions in medical centers. Research and innovative treatments give pain sufferers many new options and renewed hope. Medical professionals know that pain is a companion to most disease processes and that managing pain properly is a crucial part of recovery. Philosophically, it seems that less is more, and multidisciplinary approaches are becoming the norm. Use less narcotic medication. Have less invasive procedures. Try more strategies. Have more patience. And work with more helpers to manage the pain.

Acute pain is a familiar experience and often prevents us from really hurting ourselves. It is treated with quick fix analgesic measures until it goes away.

Chronic pain is something entirely different. It doesn't go away. The underlying injury or pathology may have long since healed. But the pain remains. When pain lasts longer than medical professionals think it should, it is considered chronic. For example, when a back-pain sufferer's discomfort lasts more than three months, it is chronic pain. Mine is going on 16 years.

If you have lived with some form of pain for a long time, you probably have your own definition for it. Having a definition is helpful. It allows us to keep our pain within mental boundaries. If we can understand it, we are better able to manage our pain instead of permitting it to control us. My definition for *chronic pain* is "severe, continuous discomfort that is very difficult to get out of mind."

It is amazing how much pain we actually have. When we *listen* to our bodies, we begin to notice what hurts and where it hurts. Life's activities generally distract us from thinking about it, so most of the time we are not bothered by our lesser aches and pains. Maybe you've observed a small child getting a minor bump on the head. He stops playing with his toys to notice the pain. He begins to cry in response. Then, just as quickly, something catches his attention. The tears evaporate. And his life returns to normal. Chronic pain is very different. The pain sufferer can't stop thinking about it. This experience forces "pain people" to look at life differently from others.

When pain refuses to go away, it isn't enough just to know what it is or even what is causing it. Much agonizing thought and prayer go into deciding how to think and feel about it. Pain people struggle to accept their pain. They struggle with expressing their pain so that others can understand them. Pain people who not only cope but ultimately thrive are those who develop a constructive personal philosophy regarding their pain experience. Or, if I may, they develop a personal *theology of their pain,* because what we think about our pain affects what we think about our God. They read and integrate the teachings of the Bible with the myriad of thoughts that are part of their personal struggle. They reflect on the life and work of Jesus for comfort and hope. And they make conscious decisions about how they intend to live under difficult, pain-filled circumstances.

I come from a German Lutheran background. We suffer well. The rules for engaging pain or any other misfortune are pretty basic: grin and bear it. But I have come to realize that, other than earning style points from Teutonic judges, there aren't many benefits to this approach to pain management. In fact, there are some real disadvantages. One disadvantage is delaying treatment that might be helpful. Another is unintentionally misleading the people around you. When I could no longer grin and bear it, I found I really didn't know what else to do. My repertoire for expressing pain was pretty limited. In public, I would grin and bear it. In private, I would be crabby or worse, especially with the people I loved the most. I now realize there are generational, cultural, ethnic, even religious factors that influence what a person thinks about pain and how a person expresses pain. In some cultures and traditions, for example, moaning is permitted. Perhaps the folks who indulge themselves in this way have discovered that wailing siphons off a lot of pain-related pressures that build up inside people like me. I confess that I thought about trying it but was afraid that I would sound like a wounded beagle.

My wife and I had the privilege of taking care of my father-in-law in our home during two episodes of serious illness. The last episode led to his death. He was a delightful man who tried to think positively, denied the seriousness of things, and never complained. If you asked him, How are you feeling? The response was always the same: Pretty good. Finally, ignored colon cancer spread to his liver and made him gravely ill. When we could no longer take adequate care of him, we took him to live in a nursing home. We visited regularly and watched his condition deteriorate with every visit. Three days before he died, we found him sitting at a dining room table, his head buried in his arms. I crouched next to him, put my hand on his shoulder, and quietly asked, "Dad, how are you doing?" It took all of the strength he had to raise his head. A string of saliva drooled from his mouth. His voice quivered in a whisper, "Pretty good." He was grinning and bearing it to the end.

Sometimes, that is all we can do. In fact, it is what we must do. I think of Job often. Sitting in misery with a body full of sores and surrounded by fools, he refused to express his pain by cursing God. His penetrating question has entered my mind many times as I have prayed for relief. "Shall we accept good from God, and not trouble?" (Job 2:10).

How we marvel at Job's submission to God's will and his patience with the people around him! But we marvel even more that Job's epic suffering was a prologue to his uttering the most hope-filled message ever spoken. Within hearing of his miserable comforters, he testified, "I know that my Redeemer lives!" How very often the pain sufferer has to help others understand his pain and cheer them up! And *that* can be a pain.

When I could no longer grin and bear it, I made the decision to resign from church work and go on long-term disability. This decision was 13 years in the making. I know it seemed rash to others. They said, "We just didn't know it was that bad." I felt like saying, "Du-u-u-h, that's because I was grinning and bearing it."

Over the years people would ask, "How's your back?" Usually, I didn't need to answer because they would go on to tell me about an episode of back pain they had experienced. When I did answer, I would say something like "It's okay" or something intended to be a little humorous: "At least I'm still vertical."

I understand human nature. People don't like complainers. None of us wants to put people off by complaining. But I now also realize that I failed to help prepare others for some of the changes my resignation would set in motion. I knew it when friends, relatives, and colleagues all asked basically the same questions: Are you sure? Are you sure it's that bad? Are you sure you are seeing the right doctor? Are you sure you are doing everything you can? Are you sure there isn't a miracle cure or a magic bullet you have overlooked? I was sure. They weren't. They weren't because I had failed to express my pain adequately.

I have decided upon this approach. I am not going to say anything unless someone asks me. Then, when they ask me, I will give them a straightforward answer.

"How's your back?"

"It is not good at all."

Then, if they ask more, I will give them details about my pain, my treatment, and my plans.

I have also decided to always tell God everything because he has asked repeatedly. In his Word he invites us again and again, "Come to me. Seek me out with a heart full of the faith I have given you. Pray without ceasing."

Three times the apostle Paul prayed for God to remove the chronic pain that stuck in his flesh like a thorn from a fire bush. And God always said, "My grace is sufficient for you, for my power is made perfect in weakness" (2 Corinthians 12:9).

To be honest, I am afraid of that answer to my prayers. I am not entirely sure what that answer will mean. I want to feel better and function better. But I do know that had God taken his thorny pain away, Paul would have been underdeveloped for the Lord's purposes. Paul would not have known the miserable joy of being broken and humbled by pain. He would not have known the miserable joy of having his ego dismantled and his self-importance disregarded by the Almighty. He would not have known the miserable joy of really being weak so that God could be strong in him and through him. Without that pain, Paul would have been useless to God and these sweet, inspired words would not have been sincere coming from him:

> Love is patient, love is kind. It does not envy, it does not boast, it is not proud. It is not rude, it is not self-seeking, it is not easily angered, it keeps no record of wrongs. Love does not delight in evil but rejoices with the truth. It always protects, always trusts, always hopes, always perseveres.
>
> 1 Corinthians 13:4-7

Chapter 2

Lightning **Strikes**

In October 1988, at the left side of the free throw lane, under the south basket, in the auxiliary gym of a large Lutheran high school in the Midwest, my life changed forever. We were gearing up for another basketball season. I decided to run layups with the kids. I went up for a rebound, twisted to the left to make an outlet pass, . . . and lightning struck. Something gave way in my lower back. It was like a cannonball hitting a rickety, old frigate broadside. Everything quivered and shook. I had never felt pain like that in my life and had no idea what it was.

After a brief pause and noble effort not to let on that anything was wrong, I concluded that I had pulled a muscle or something. *I'll just run it off,* I thought. I kept going, and so did the pain. I made it home, got undressed, and crawled into bed.

The next morning the pain was worse. Every move resulted in excruciating spasms. I couldn't twist or bend. My wife literally had to dress me. She said, "You really shouldn't go to school today. You should see a doctor."

I said, "I have never missed a day yet; I am not going to start now."

She said, "Okay, you stupid man. But you will be sorry."

She was right. I have been sorry since 1988. And I have long since repented of arrogance masquerading as servanthood. God didn't need me that day like I thought he did. In fact, I found out some 17 years later that he didn't need me at all in the way I thought he did.

Over the next several weeks, the spasms quieted down and the pain in my lower back disappeared. All I really noticed was tightness in my right leg. A little bothersome, but I could handle it. Slowly and steadily it got worse. The tightness gave way to cramping pain. I had trouble sitting or standing for any length of time.

I finally started going to doctors. They prescribed very nice pain pills and issued dire warnings that I should stay in bed for several weeks because I might have herniated a disc in my back. Stay in bed? They just didn't understand. I had tons of commitments to my wife and three small children, my teaching, graduate school, and other church work. I had to keep going.

And keep going is what I did, until one decisive weekend.

I went with a group to make a presentation at a church conference in another state. I rode along with several others in a big station wagon. On the way I sat in the seat like normal people do. I had to fidget a lot, but I made it. I came home lying in the back with all of the baggage and curled up in a ball of pain. That night my wife took me to the emergency room. The ER doctor gave me more pills and a referral to a neurological surgeon.

By the time I got in to see the doctor, I could hardly function. I couldn't stand long enough to shave. I couldn't sit long enough to eat. I could barely get out of bed. The pain shot down my right leg, through my calf, and into my foot. Unless I was lying down, it would build to the point that I thought I was going to pass out. That has always been the pattern of my back pain. I rarely felt any discomfort in my back where the real problem was located. The pain would instead radiate along nerve pathways and wreak havoc on my lower extremities. (C. S. Lewis said that pain is God's megaphone. *Jason, can you hear me now?* "Yes, Lord, your servant is listening.") I was at a point where I didn't care what the doctor did. Fortunately, I would be seeing a young surgeon who cared very much what he did.

My doctor is the kind of surgeon every back patient should have. He is very conservative in his approach. In his view, surgery is a last resort. And he is very skilled when he finally does operate. That was the approach he took with me. He ordered two weeks of complete bed rest. To help me comply he prescribed high doses of Valium, ibuprofen, and Tylenol with codeine, which I took three times a day. He was hoping to get me to relax. Keeping me inactive would cause the suspected bulging disc to loosen its grip on my life. It didn't. And then I had a new and wicked ailment as a side effect of all the pills and inactivity. Something like liquid drain cleaner was required to remedy this.

My physician sent me to physical therapy sessions in the hope that gentle manipulation and ultrasound heat treatments might help. It felt good while they were doing it. But it didn't change my condition. He ordered X rays, CT scans, MRIs. These tests indicated that the L4-L5 disc space was a little narrow. He sent me for injections in that epidural space, hoping that the steroid would provide some relief and settle things down. Finally, he sent me for a myelogram. It clearly showed a protruding disc. Later he would discover that that "stinkin' little disc" had slammed itself into the sciatic nerve root and had wedged it against some bone. It wasn't going to budge.

After several weeks of trying everything conservative, my doctor said that I was a good candidate for surgery. Now I hadn't been in a hospital since my birth. I had never had any kind of surgery. I had read the horror stories and heard dire warnings to avoid back surgery at all costs. But by this time, if he had said, "We need to amputate everything from the waist down," I would have said, "Let's go."

Over the years a number of people with back pain have contacted me to talk about my experience and to gather information to help them make a decision regarding surgery. I usually tell them to avoid surgery if at all possible. I tell them that in my experience, back surgery doesn't eliminate pain, it just changes pain. I tell them that the body has a capacity to heal itself, and most people that have severe episodes of back pain will recover nicely without surgery. I tell them to be very patient and give it lots of time. And I tell them that they will know when they should have surgery because the pain of body and soul has sucked any joy out of their lives. When that happens, back surgery might be the last and best hope for some joy to return. But they should prepare themselves for what could be a miserable kind of joy.

It was right before Easter in 1989 that I had a lumbar laminectomy/discectomy. An incision of a couple of inches was made in my lower back. The skin, muscle, and other tissue was exposed and spread. A small piece of the bone protecting the spinal column was removed. The sciatic nerve was very carefully set aside. And the offending disc material was removed. The remaining disc was poked several times to form scar tissue. This would make the remaining disc tough enough to support the vertebrae above it. That was the theory.

I was actually looking forward to going under the anesthetic because I knew that for a while I would feel no pain. When I came out of the anesthetic, the pain that had brought me there was gone. I was ecstatic. Of course, I still felt pain from the surgery, but the leg pain had all but vanished.

The first night several nurses helped me out of bed and managed to get me to walk. I was a little shaky, but I could tell that walking was a good thing. The more I walked, the better I felt; and the looser the muscles became, the stronger my back seemed. After a while I was able to get up by myself to walk, especially at night when I couldn't sleep. The poor guy in the bed next to me had the same surgery the day before I did. He still wasn't up walking around. Now there was a competitive element, and I was winning. The staff praised me for my progress. I was released ahead of schedule, went home, and walked some more. I was highly motivated to get better—to get back to normal. That was a very special Easter. Jesus lives! And I was better. I wish this story had ended right then and there. But it doesn't. And I realize now that, for me, new chapters will continue to be written as long as I live.

I began to settle back into a routine—what most people would think of as a normal way of living. Some lingering muscle stiffness in my lower back and buttocks remained, but I was able to return to my life and my work with energy and enthusiasm.

After a year's time, I began to notice some changes. Slowly, insidiously, the pain was intensifying. And now it shot down both legs. I exercised more, stretched more. But week after week I could tell it was getting worse. I tried a lot of things to avoid returning to my surgeon: chiropractic treatment, acupuncture, pharmaceuticals. Nothing relieved the pain. I knew in my gut that I was facing a worst-case scenario—a back surgery that was not holding up. This was a sucker punch to the stomach. I had just accepted the position to serve as principal and administrator of a high school that had fallen on hard times. I needed to be at the top of my game. Instead, I would go into my new job with severe pain and a deteriorating condition. I was beyond depressed.

After getting some second opinions, I returned to my surgeon. Once again, he was welcoming and encouraging. Once again, he put me through a series of conservative measures. But as the weeks wore on, the pain got worse and I got more desperate. Finally, and reluctantly, he suggested that a fusion might give me some relief. I knew this would be major surgery. And I knew the prognosis would be guarded at best. But there was no joy in my life, and I was ready once again to try anything for some measure of relief from the pain.

My first back surgery had taken one and a half hours. The second time around, I was on the table for more than six hours. This was not a tune-up. It was a major overhaul of my lumbar spine. The incision ran from my tailbone to the middle of my back. After doing what had to be done to reveal the spine, an awful lot of bone, disc material, and other tissue was removed from the three lower levels of my spine. Along each side of the area the bone was scraped until it bled. New bleeding bone was then grafted from the crest of my pelvis and laid along the prepared area. Then, to hold it all in place while the bone graft grew solid, six large screws were installed into the vertebral blocks and four plates were bolted on. What once had been a flexible lower back was now rock solid.

As soon as I came out of the anesthetic, I knew my situation was very different from the aftermath of my first surgery. For one thing, the surgical pain was much more severe because the surgery had been so extensive. When they log-rolled me over in bed, pain radiated down my legs and my feet cramped severely. After a few days they got me up to walk. Remembering how helpful that was from the first surgery, I tried to repeat my winning performance. Not this time. The more I walked, the more intense the pain became. I was not pain-free by any means. Time would prove that I would never be pain-free again. But I could tell that this time the pain was different. Time would also prove that the pain was reduced by the surgery and would become more manageable with each passing year. But the improvement was so subtle that I couldn't perceive it from day to day. I can only look back in retrospect and see that I could tolerate similar events better after my second surgery. In my case God used very slow progress to give me something that I thought was for people who really didn't have much to do: patience.

The second surgery permitted me to continue to serve God and my church for 13 joy-filled years. Although pain was my constant companion, I enjoyed the privilege of serving as a teacher, counselor, high school principal, church consultant, and denominational administrator. And I was able to live a fulfilling family life and personal life. As my condition deteriorated, I made accommodations. I spent two years doing all of my "sitting" work standing at a raised platform. When I could no longer bear to sit or stand, and there was no joy, just misery, I finally resigned and went on disability.

My faithful surgeon has always taken a very deliberate approach to my condition. He referred me to an excellent pain specialist who tried everything he knew to give me some relief. And he did, at least temporarily. I have undergone facet joint injections in the space above my fusion. The short-term relief from the searing leg pain served as a clue, telling him that the joint above my fusion was the culprit. This is not a surprise to people who understand the classic progression of post-fusion back failure. The fusion locked the lowest, largest, and strongest spinal levels together. As a result, the level above the fusion had to take over the weight-bearing and movement functions. It did this for 13 years. Oh, it complained plenty over those years. But, all things considered, it did a pretty good job.

In an effort to provide longer lasting relief, the pain specialist performed two rounds of radio-frequency nerve ablation at the levels above the fusion. Using a needle and radio waves, he burned out the sensory nerve that carried the pain signal from the facet joint to the brain. This helped sustain relief, especially from my leg pain. To address the back and buttocks pain, he administered a caudal epidural injection and an epidural injection in the space above the fusion. Again, the relief was short term, but it confirmed that the major source of my pain continued to be that degenerated level above the fusion.

As much as my surgeon and I would like to avoid another surgery, I think we are reaching a consensus that it may be the last best hope for some joy to return to my life. So, while I am desperate for relief and some joy to return to my life, I am prepared for the fact that it is likely to be miserable joy once again.

Back on May 1, 1990, when the diagnosis had confirmed that my first back surgery was not holding up, I was discouraged and frightened. I turned to the powerful Word of God for hope and comfort. Not knowing exactly where I wanted to go in Scripture, I stumbled upon Hebrews chapter 12. What wonderful words the Holy Spirit inspired there! It was as if the words of that chapter were meant just for me. I made a note in the margin documenting the date. I read. I cried. I prayed. I placed my hope in these powerful words: "Therefore, since we are surrounded by such a great cloud of witnesses, let us throw off everything that hinders and the sin that so easily entangles, and let us run with perseverance the race marked out for us" (verse 1).

Lord, forgive my lack of trust and my fear. If this is the race you have marked out for me, let me run it faithfully. I am encouraged by the recollection of those believers who have run even tougher races in the past and who have persevered. As you enabled them to run this race, please stay close to my side.

"Let us fix our eyes on Jesus, the author and perfecter of our faith, who for the joy set before him endured the cross, . . . and sat down at the right hand of the throne of God" (verse 2).

O Lord, I cannot imagine what Jesus went through. He suffered torture, death, and hell itself. He did it for the joy of redeeming me and all people. He did it for the joy of returning to the glorious right hand of his heavenly Father. What miserable joy for him! Let me look on him in faith and look forward to being with him in heaven.

"Endure hardship as discipline; God is treating you as sons" (verse 7).

Lord, thank you for making me your child. What grace is experienced in being your son and heir! I accept this very tough time as part of your plan to make me an even better son.

"No discipline seems pleasant at the time, but painful. Later on, however, it produces a harvest of righteousness and peace for those who have been trained by it" (verse 11).

Lord, I've got to be honest with you. I don't like this one bit. I was hoping for a more pleasant life. I also have to be honest with myself; you are not done with me yet. Apparently there is a lot of room for growth. Let me learn quickly. Train my mind, my heart, and my spirit so that my life gives a clear testimony to what you have done for me in Christ.

"Therefore, strengthen your feeble arms and weak knees. 'Make level paths for your feet,' so that the lame may not be disabled, but rather healed" (verses 12,13).

Lord, you picture a spiritual journey for me. How weak and inadequate is every member of my being. The pathway is lumpy, and there is a risk that I will stumble or cause someone else to stumble. Smooth out this path by strengthening my faith through your Holy Word. Help me set a good example for others whose lives also limp. But for me, Lord, this spiritual journey is also physical. There is real and actual weakness in my knees and my legs. I am disabled. Lord, please strengthen my feeble arms and weak knees. Provide enough healing that I might find joy.

For Jesus' sake . . .

Chapter 3

Dark Places

It is frightening where the mind can go. Hidden in the wrinkles of the brain are the seeds for some pretty noxious thoughts. It doesn't take much for those thoughts to grow and overtake a healthy frame of mind. The mind is one of the greatest of all God's gifts given to human beings. We don't just have a brain; we have a mind. We are capable of rational thoughts and irrational thoughts. We can solve problems or fixate on things we have no business thinking about. We can reminisce about the past with fondness or dwell on past mistakes. We can anticipate events and plan for the future or look down the road with fear and dread. None of us fully understands the power God has packed into our mental being—power that can be used for better and for worse. No doubt that is why God inspired Paul to write, "Whatever is true, whatever is noble, whatever is right, whatever is pure, whatever is lovely, whatever is admirable—if anything is excellent or praiseworthy—think about such things" (Philippians 4:8).

Battling chronic pain demands incredible mental discipline. And God has given us the ability to exercise that discipline. Our thoughts are the launching pad for emotions and actions. They play off one another. We honestly have to work at keeping our thoughts in check. That difficult work is enabled with Bible reading. Through the very words of God, the Holy Spirit sheds the light of God's love and the hope of his promises into the dark corners of our deflated spirits. Rigorous prayer is our access to God's ears and permits us to wrestle with our thoughts and feelings out loud. We can hear what we are saying to God. We vent what we need to vent. We praise him and plead for his healing and the ability to accept his will. The company of family and friends is essential to expose us to the thinking of others. Their ways of looking at our situation and their words of encouragement nudge our thoughts out of their dark silos. Unless we think about our thinking and manage our thoughts, our minds will wander off into some pretty dark places. Our feelings and actions will follow.

In the late 1960s Elisabeth Kübler-Ross did groundbreaking work on dealing with trauma and loss. Her theory has stood the test of time and is effectively summarized in five stages: *denial, anger, bargaining, depression,* and *acceptance.* Most people will deal with most serious changes in their lives by making their way through these stages. It is helpful for folks to know that having these thoughts is common. Therapists have found this scheme useful in helping clients work through the loss of loved ones and other very important events. I recognize these thoughts in my own grief over the loss of my physical well-being and my career. But I have also found that living with chronic pain invites many other thoughts and feelings that don't follow any tidy progression. These are the dark places of my mind.

Frustration is a dark, enslaving place. I have been filled with it. At times I want to explode. It is so frustrating to wake every morning hoping against hope that when my feet hit the floor, the pressure won't build and the pain will be diminished. It's the same day after day. Day after day I want to do things. Day after day I try to do things. And day after day I am sidelined by pain. That ticking sound you hear is the bomb inside of me; it is waiting to go off. I haven't seen 50 years yet. I have lots of things I would like to do before my life is over. To others I appear as I always have. All indications are that I am healthy otherwise. There is still energy in my mind and fight in my spirit. But there is the wall of pain. I hit it every single day. Acquaintances don't see the pain. Without a lengthy explanation, they don't understand what gives. My life seems to be one of missed opportunity. And that is very frustrating.

Anger is a dark, destructive place. It is frustration escaping through a crack in self-control. For males in our culture, anger is the emotion of choice. When we don't know what else to be, we become angry. For a male with chronic pain, that anger is loaded on a hair trigger. Sometimes it doesn't take much to fire off a few rounds. Sadly, it is usually those we love the most that get hit. It has been well said that hurting people hurt people. I have admitted to my family that there are days I want to be mad at something. There are days I am looking for a fight. I have assured them I don't want to be mad at them. But they often end up being collateral damage in this terrible war against pain. They experience sharp words and impatience over something insignificant. That is nothing more than the shrapnel of anger. I am angry at the pain. I am angry with myself for not somehow avoiding this nightmare. I don't think I am angry with God, but there are days I don't feel like talking to him.

Envy is a dark, puny place. I am embarrassed to admit to it. It took me totally by surprise. I never thought I was an envious person. But I go there sometimes. When I see fit and able-bodied people enjoying life, I am envious. I would never wish pain or illness on anyone. I just wish I could sit, or stand, or move like they can. I am envious of the contestants who can bend over and spin that giant wheel on that game show. They can give it a mighty spin. If I were doing it, I would have to crouch next to it and give it a feeble push. I am envious of the men who can sit on a wooden bench with their wives to watch the sun set over the ocean. I would have to bring a cushion and couldn't stay very long. Somehow that is not part of the romance of the moment. I am envious of people who can go to ball games, attend concerts, and sit in the boat all day to fish. I am envious of the people around me in church who are paying better attention than I am because pain isn't making them wish it was over.

Bitterness is a dark and acrid place. It is the result of stewing in the juices of one's deepest disappointments. My wife called me on it. She said, "Jason, you are becoming a bitter, old man." She was right. There was bitterness within me. And it was changing who I am. It was changing how I respond to just about everything. It was discoloring how I saw the past and what I expected in the future. I was bitter over working hard for 28 years, getting to a position of great responsibility, and then having to give it up. I was bitter that while this gnawed at me daily, others seemed to get over it pretty quickly. I was bitter thinking that people were interested in me when I had something to offer, but not now. I was bitter that life's train was leaving the station and I couldn't get on it. The bitterness expressed itself in a few choice words of self-pity that came from seeing myself as an undeserving victim. Bitterness was changing me from being a positive man to becoming a negative man. I don't want to be that man.

Isolation is a dark and lonely place. Somehow, when we need to be with people the most, we want to be with them the least. Part of it is a function of pain. It is hard to engage in the pleasantries of socializing when you need to go lie down so the spasms in your back and legs will quiet down. It is also a function of circumstances. Boy, does a house get quiet after everyone is off to work and school and you're alone wondering, *What can I do to pass the time today?* People who are in pain often don't feel like being with others. It takes too much energy to fight the pain and hold up your end of a conversation at the same time. It takes so much concentration to ignore the pain and show interest in the things that interest others. It takes so much endurance to get through events that it just isn't worth going. I hate being alone. And I hate going where people are and trying to do the things they are doing.

The worst isolation of all is from God. Is he leaving me or am I leaving him? I wonder along with David, "Why, O LORD, do you stand far off?" (Psalm 10:1). But sometimes I am the one standing far off, from God and everyone else. Being alone with thoughts from dark places is unhealthy in every way.

Despair is a dark and dangerous place. It is an emotional and spiritual free fall. Day after day, week after week, year after year of pain poke too many holes in hope. It can't float anymore. Despair leaks in. So does Satan. It is frightening where the mind will go. Especially when Satan uses pain to make the unthinkable, thinkable. Despair makes pain worse. The brain must squirt out different chemicals when we are despairing than when we are hoping. Pain under the influence of hope can be survived, even overcome. But pain weighed down by despair can destroy us. I didn't think about ending my life for very long. But I did pray that God would. I don't want to be irreverent here, but there were times I would not have objected if God had dispatched a Peterbilt with my name scrolled across its massive chrome grille.

These are my dark places. If you have pain in your life, you have dark places too. They may be similar, or they may be very different. But please be aware that these are places our minds take us. Our conversations within ourselves about our pain and situation create a snowball of thoughts rumbling downhill. This is an oversimplification. But it is also true. We think ourselves into dark places. We have to think ourselves out of them. Many of us will be able to think ourselves out of them on our own. Some of us may need the help of a pastor, a friend, or even a therapist. But it is essential that we think ourselves out of them.

Philosopher René Descartes figured this out. His announcement is classic: "I think, therefore I am." Perhaps he was echoing Solomon's wisdom: "As [a man] thinketh in his heart, so is he" (Proverbs 23:7 KJV). We will not be able to think ourselves out of our dark places without encountering divine thinking.

We encounter divine thinking in God's Word.

Chapter 11 of Romans is a difficult passage. It describes how people enter and leave God's family. We are given a look into things that are really none of our concern. The apostle Paul characterizes the justice and mercy of God as he lops unfaithful branches off his family tree and graciously attaches healthy new ones. With this Paul gives us a look at God's way of thinking. "Consider therefore the kindness and sternness of God: sternness to those who fell, but kindness to you, provided that you continue in his kindness" (verse 22). This isn't double-talk but a description of the Christian's touch-and-go with God. It is God's kindness that enables us to continue in his kindness. It is God's faithfulness to us that enables us to remain faithful to him. It is Christ's death for us that gives us the desire to live for him.

Paul closes the chapter with a beautiful doxology to the way God thinks:

> Oh, the depth of the riches of the wisdom and knowledge of God! How unsearchable his judgments, and his paths beyond tracing out! "Who has known the mind of the Lord? Or who has been his counselor?" "Who has ever given to God, that God should repay him?"
>
> For from him and through him and to him are all things. To him be the glory forever! Amen.
>
> Romans 11:33-36

In essence, Paul is saying, "Don't even try to figure it all out. You can't. But know this, there is no *God bypass* on life's road." It is all from him and to him and through him—

even our pain. God's thinking about us is embedded in his love for us. He thinks of us joined to the recollection of what his Son has done for us. God owes us nothing and gives us everything. The way out of our dark places is to peer into the depth of God's love in Jesus Christ.

That is how Paul could go on:

> Therefore, I urge you, brothers, in view of God's mercy, to offer your bodies as living sacrifices, holy and pleasing to God—this is your spiritual act of worship. Do not conform any longer to the pattern of this world, but be transformed by the *renewing of your mind.* Then you will be able to test and approve what God's will is—his good, pleasing and perfect will.
>
> Romans 12:1,2 (italics added)

God's mercy changes everything, including our thinking. Keeping the mercy of God at the forefront of our thoughts is the beacon of hope that leads us out of those dark places. God wants our pain-filled bodies, even more than we do. He wants our pain-filled lives, even more than we do. He wants us to give it up, pain and all, for him and to him and through him. This kind of total dependency is the ultimate act of worship. It is only possible when we think less about ourselves, less about our pain, and much more about Christ's suffering, death, and resurrection. It is through Jesus that God has called us out of darkness into his wonderful light. We may never be healed, but hear this well: *We can be transformed!* We can be transformed by the renewing of our minds as his Holy Spirit brings God's Word and his promises to bear in our desperate lives. And in the end that will prove to be even better. It reintroduces joy into our lives at a whole new and wonderful level. It does so by changing the question from, What in the world is God doing *to* me? to, What in *this* world does God still want to do *through* me?

Chapter 4

Disabled for What?

The darkest place I have ever been in is disability. *Disability.* I hate the sight of the word. I hate the sound of the word. I hate all of the implications of the word. Going on disability was the most discouraging experience of my life. For months I dwelt on all the hopeless consequences of being *dissed* of ability. Every day I struggled to answer the question, "What has become of *me?*"

By the time I reached middle age, I had a pretty well-defined self-concept. Years of family life, education, work, promotions, successes, failures, recoveries, and feedback from others provided the building blocks for my identity. By middle age I had a litany of ways to finish every thought that begins with *I am*. I became comfortable with them. They rolled off my tongue effortlessly whenever someone asked, "Who are you?" or "What do you do?" Then a lousy word of ten little letters erased them all. The *D*-word. And every understanding of what I am was blown away with the chilling blast of facing what I am not.

Going on disability necessitated lots of changes in my personal life and our family life. We had to sell our home and move to a more modest house in a new neighborhood. I dreaded meeting the very nice people who lived around us. I knew what they were going to ask: "So, Jason, what do you do?"

How we define ourselves is not only what we do but also how others size us up. Asking that question is the informal background check we conduct with new people we meet. The answer provides a gateway for more conversation and maybe even friendship. That is why it is so hard to answer, "Nothing."

Or, worse yet, to launch into a tirade explaining the hard-luck story of one's life: "Yeah, I used to be a teacher and leader in the church. I used to help kids and families and churches. I used to be a husband that could go for walks with his wife and enjoy an evening out. I used to be a dad that could roughhouse with his children and play catch with them in the backyard. I used to be a guy that family and friends could count on to help them when they needed it. I used to love doing home improvement projects. I couldn't wait to go fishing. I used to daydream about having grandchildren and imagine the kind of fun-loving grandfather I wanted to be. But I am none of those things now. No, I am none of those things. You see, I am *disabled*."

What makes chronic pain so cruel is that it is an invisible disability. In many cases it is not self-evident. No one else can see it unless the sufferers let their guard down. People who meet pain people are not restrained by the social mores that cause them to deal sensitively with an amputee or kindly with a person locked in the perpetual childhood of Downs Syndrome. In order for them to know what your disability is, you have to tell them. And it is perturbing to reiterate, I am just not the person I used to be. Believe me, anyone who has ever gone from being able-bodied to becoming disabled has heard the gurgling sound of his or her personhood being flushed away. The emotions involved are way beyond self-pity. How does one adjust to the evacuation of every understanding of who he is? And to the reader who might be inclined to say, "You just shouldn't feel that way," please don't add insult to injury.

Disability is a matter of degrees. We are all disabled to some degree ever since sin entered the world. None of us can see perfectly or hear perfectly. None of us can think without some kind of brain wave interference. We remember less than we could. We move less than we should. The list can go on. Every hitch in our stride is a little reminder that we are all less than God intended us to be. And we will remain that way until God replaces these disabled bodies with those new bodies that will be like the glorious body of our risen and ascended Lord Jesus.

For many of us though, heaven may be a long way off. In the meantime we must learn to live with disability.

Learning to live with disability raises so many questions. The answers are oh, so illusive. Learning to live with disability may mean that just knowing the questions is enough. So much of life really isn't about having all the answers. It is about knowing the right questions.

What am I here for? That is a really great question. It hints at its own answer. There is a reason we are here. If there were no reason, we wouldn't be here. If God were done with us, we would be dead. Life itself is strong evidence that there is still a reason for our being on this earth. What am I here for? The question matters. It drives us to strive to answer it. It drives us to discover the gifts and talents God has given us. It drives us to learn, grow, and grapple with the purpose for our existence. It is a great question, and we never answer it completely. We find partial answers in each stage and transition of our lives. But it always remains a great question.

For months I continued to ask that great question: What am I here for? But it no longer sounded like a great question. It was different now. The little voice in my head that asked it sounded pretty defeated. The tone of the question suggested that there was no answer. I heard it with a hollow sigh. And then it occurred to me. I needed a new question. Don't get me wrong; *What am I here for?* is always a great question. But it wasn't doing much for me. A new question changed everything for me. The new question was *What am I disabled for?*

That question also hints at its own answer. It supposes that I have been disabled for a purpose. Now the tone of the little voice is not defeated but curious. At times it is even energized. What am I disabled for? It suggests that a turning is occurring in my life. It suggests that for some reason God interrupted the life I had. I must be honest. I have no idea what the answer is . . . yet. But knowing that this is the right question has been a breakthrough. It has brought some joy back into my life. It is still miserable joy, but it's also eager joy. I am eager to see where God will lead me. And I am more ready to accept the answer.

I just know I am not the first disabled person to ask that question. When polio crippled Franklin Delano Roosevelt, he must have asked, "What am I disabled for?" Perhaps he never fully understood the answer. But his disability gave him even greater ability to inspire and lead our nation during a difficult time in its history.

When the brilliant mind of Helen Keller broke free from its dark and silent prison, she must have asked herself, "What am I disabled for?" Her sense of the answer enabled her to be a stirring advocate that changed forever the way the world looks at people with disabilities.

Stevie Wonder and Ronnie Milsap have never seen the notes. But they make music as well as anyone. Their ability to play and sing has delighted millions. They are legends in the music industry. That is what they were disabled for.

The list could go on. Disabled heroes are all around us. Some have celebrity and others are celebrities in smaller circles. Some days I am able to take short walks in our new neighborhood. I have walked past a little house with a large deck on the front. On nice days, a woman in a wheelchair sits on that deck. At first I didn't look at her long because I didn't want to seem like I was staring at her. Eventually I waved, and she waved back with great exuberance. Next I greeted her, and she responded with one of the most cheerful voices I have ever heard. Someday, I hope to have the courage to go over to her deck and engage in a conversation. I want to know her story. I want to know how she came to understand what she was disabled for. It is clear that her legs don't work and that she is dependent on wheels. I have a hunch God also gave her wings. "Those who hope in the LORD will renew their strength. They will soar on wings like eagles; they will run and not grow weary, they will walk and not be faint" (Isaiah 40:31). How could she have such a soaring spirit without wings?

Jeremiah was not God's most cheerful prophet. The circumstances of his life and ministry were desperate. Some of God's people had to be carried into captivity to learn what God wanted to teach them. Others remained behind in a Promised Land turned desolate. Depression ran rampant. Most of the time the best Jeremiah could do was raise questions. "Why does the way of the wicked prosper?" he wondered. "How long will the land lie parched?" A clear answer from God was slow in coming. His people had to be content with the questions they had and the promise that God had answers. He assured them: "'For I know the plans I have for you,' declares the LORD, 'plans to prosper you and not to harm you, plans to give you hope and a future'" (Jeremiah 29:11).

Chapter 5

God's Sense of **Timing**

In a popular Country song, Sara Evans sings of a young woman struggling to find her place in life. As the tear-jerking tale is told, a line is thrown out to reconcile all the twists and turns of her life. She sings, "God has a funny sense of timing." This is the conclusion when the song's unfortunate heroine becomes pregnant and gives birth at a very inopportune time. But what a gift her baby turns out to be! One moral of the story is that bad timing to us is right timing for God.

It takes maturity to recognize this. Interpreting life according to the will of God is an advanced skill of veteran Christians. In order to be able to look back with some sense of perspective, one has to get down the road a piece. In order to be able to trust God's sense of timing, one has to be able to reflect on it over a lifetime. God's funny sense of timing is appreciated by the student, forced to change schools against her will only to have the best experience of her life. God's funny sense of timing is discovered by the man, laid off from his job of many years only to find the career of a lifetime. When we appreciate God's funny sense of timing, each quirky turn of events causes us to ask ourselves, "I wonder what he's got in mind this time?"

Actually, one could argue that God has no sense of timing. Time itself is his creation. For some reason he felt we would need it, but he doesn't. God *is*, from eternity to eternity. He began in timelessness and exists in timelessness. The place where God lives has no deadlines, just destinies. Your destiny and my destiny are part of God's wonderful sense of timing. Your destiny and my destiny have been made sure by the suffering, death, and resurrection of Jesus Christ, who left his comfort zone in a boundless universe to live for a while among us in the restrictive corridor of time. Your destiny and my destiny are not part of an amorphous lava flow that we just happen to have gotten caught in. Your destiny and my destiny are the result of God's very careful ordering of the events of our lives, marking time for each of us.

My wife and I enjoyed God's funny sense of timing when our son Jordan came along. We were heading toward middle age at a pretty good clip. The son we had come to accept as the baby of our family was eight years old. The house was filling up with all of the paraphernalia of two daughters in their teenage years. It seemed like a good time to have a garage sale. The crib went quickly. So did the high chair, the changing table, the little plastic bathtub, and the toys that went with it. Every last artifact of the baby stage of life was grabbed up by bargain hunters and carried away in mini vans to more appropriate homes.

Besides, we had other things to be concerned about. We had moved to a new community. I was working at a new position as a Lutheran high school principal and facing a second major back surgery. Having another child was the furthest thing from our minds. But it was not far from God's mind, because his sense of timing is intentional. Nothing happens by accident with him. This "whoops" in our family planning was something God had thought about, planned for, and brought about at just the right time.

When Nancy realized she might be expecting, she spent some weeks in denial before breaking the news to me. I needed more evidence than just the internal knowing of a lady who had been pregnant several times before. So we got one of those home pregnancy tests. There was high drama in the moment. We stared in silence at the confirming color of the test. Then we looked at each other. Then we looked back at the test. Then we looked back at each other and just laughed. The laughter relieved a lot of tension. And, sure, the laughter was an expression of our joy. And we laughed because we recognized the irony of the situation.

First of all, how would our older children react? This would come as a total surprise. It would bring all of those carefully told tales of the birds and the bees a little too close to home for their liking. It is one thing to understand God's gift of sexuality in the abstract, something engaged in by nameless and faceless people in the crowd. It is quite another thing to realize that people you eat supper with each day are doing it. They had been at the garage sale. They had witnessed all the baby stuff being adopted into new families. The conclusion was obvious. No more babies in this house. A conscious decision.

And then what about family, friends, and people in the new community we served? Everyone knew I had a really bad back. Everyone knew I was scheduled for a major surgery. Having a bad back and having a baby would bring a reaction. It was universal. Each clever person's commentary on the news was the same: I thought you had a bad back? It was especially embarrassing among my high school students. I was happy they were comfortable with their new principal and found him approachable. They didn't shy away from offering their take on the situation. Even what I think they intended as compliments made me blush. One senior boy said, "Mr. Nelson, we thought you were marginally cool to begin with; now we think you are awesome." I just prayed he wouldn't elaborate.

Never once did we regret God's sense of timing. The excitement of our older children was overflowing. Jordan became the apple of all of their eyes. They ran home from school to hold him and see what new baby tricks he had learned that day. He was a special gift for a mom who is as good with babies as anyone. And he provided a lifeline forward for a father who needed it badly.

As I was recovering from the fusion I had in 1990, my doctor's instructions included, "No bending or twisting at the waist. And don't lift anything heavier than a gallon of milk." I asked him for how long those instructions applied. He said, "For the rest of your life."

That last rule hurt the most. I knew there was a pretty good chance that someday our new baby would weigh more than a gallon of milk. I wanted to be the same kind of father with him that I had been to the older children. I wanted to take my turn holding him in church or carrying him out when he needed to be carried out. I wanted to toss him gently in the air and make him giggle and laugh. I wanted him to know the smell of my skin up close and the tickle of my whiskers. I didn't want him to grow up with a dim recollection of a father who was a weak shadow in the background. In the end, none of this may have mattered to him. But it desperately mattered to me. There was only one thing to do. I broke the rule.

No, I wasn't foolish enough to risk serious injury to an already dysfunctional back. But I made a conscious decision to look and act as normal with Jordan as possible and to find things that we could do together. I made a decision to live my life and to live it with him. The things we did together proved to be the beginning of a relationship of complementary companionship. I couldn't bend at the waist to drop seeds in the garden, but I could hoe a row. And Jordan was just the right size to place those tiny seeds in their final resting places with his little fingers to await their resurrection as the fruit-producing plants from which they came. As time went on we wrestled on the floor, played catch, and did most of the things dads and sons should do. And when I had to turn in earlier than most people because I couldn't stand or sit anymore, he would climb in bed next to me and we would sing "B-I-B-L-E," "Gospel Light," "Wise Man—Foolish Man," "Jesus Loves Me," and other songs of faith, while lying flat on our backs. And we would do all of the hand gestures with energy. I needed to do what was developmentally appropriate for a growing Christian boy.

When I became disabled, Jordan became a teenager. And I came to realize that God's got a very practical sense of timing. Certainly Jordan's worth in our family is way beyond being cheap help. But the blessing of having him around is not lost on me. To have such a strong, cooperative, and competent son still at home after the others have gone is a gift God gave us 13 years ago. We just didn't fully realize how rich a blessing it would be at the time. God's got a funny, intentional, and practical sense of timing.

The worst year of my life was 2003; I hit bottom that summer. There were so many losses and so many uncertainties. I was forced to resign the ministry of a lifetime. We went through the nerve-racking process of applying for disability income, which, if granted, would reduce our household income significantly. We had to sell our home within a tight time frame and buy down in order to avoid having a financial train wreck. We had to place my father-in-law in a nursing home and have power of attorney over his health and affairs. We had to move my elderly and dependent parents out of a home we had provided for them for many years so that it could be sold. And I had to do much of this with searing pain radiating down my back, buttocks, and legs. If there hadn't been so much to do, I might have given up. But God has an intrepid sense of timing. He kept me moving out of necessity. Busi*ness* was a good distraction for a man who was close to despair and couldn't possibly see anything bright in the future. And then he provided a most wonderful sign. At least that is how I took it.

Our first daughter was expecting our first grandchild that summer. It was the solitary event that we all looked forward to. We are a close family anyway, and the arrival of another generation to love in Christ was loaded with anticipation. The due date was sometime in early July. It came and went. The anticipation for that blessed event just grew. Then we finally got the call. Late in the evening on

July 21, 2003, Abigail Katherine was born. She was born on my birthday. My first grandchild was born on my very own birthday. She was born on my birthday at the worst time during the worst year of my life. What a birthday present!

Now I know that our God is a God of signs and wonders. Many times they are there in the little things. I confess that I have never looked for too many of them outside of those recorded in his Word. But I immediately grabbed hold of this one. I absolutely delighted in the divine coincidence of Abby's birth with mine. It somehow seemed very providential. The summer Abby celebrated her 2nd birthday I celebrated my 51st, on the very same day. I know that I am not the only grandparent to share a birthday with a grandchild. Those who do have special bonds and memorable celebrations. That is all good for them too. But, believe me, I deeply inhaled every fragrance of that baby. They were "smelling salts" awakening a new consciousness and a renewed hope. Where there is life, there is hope. And I hope and pray to be granted the opportunity to be the kind of grandfather to Abby that I have always wanted to be.

One day I went for a walk down to the lake near our home. A young mom was there in the park with her two small children and one very large dog. The little boy was in a stroller and the little girl looked to be about three. All the little girl wanted to do was go out on the pier and look for some fish. The mom couldn't go because she had to hold on to the little boy and the big dog.

I said, "I'll help you find some fish." When I pointed one out to her, she crouched down and briefly glanced into the water.

Then, without a segue but with pinpoint relevance, she looked up at me and said, "My grandpa takes me fishing."

My heart melted. How I yearn for Abby to someday be able to tell someone something similar.

God has a very personalized sense of timing. He knows just what each of us needs and exactly when he or she needs it. Nothing happens by accident with God. His scheduling is not nonchalant. It is purposeful and personalized. My dear hurting friend, please know this: *Everything is right on schedule for you.*

God's sense of timing was never more apropos than when he sent his Son. Doubt among believers must have run rampant after months, years, decades, centuries, and millennia spent in waiting for the Hope of Israel to be revealed. "But when the time had fully come, God sent his Son, born of a woman, born under law, to redeem those under law that we might receive the full rights of sons" (Galatians 4:4,5). God sent Jesus at just the right time. World civilization had come far enough along but not too far along. The roads were good enough for travel but not so good as to eliminate challenging journeys. Medicine existed, but diseases still needed miraculous healing. Justice was established, but verdicts were not always fair, especially for an itinerant teacher from Galilee. Believers clung to inspired promises rolled up in flimsy scrolls, but they might not have held on for much longer if the Word had not become flesh. This was just the right time. Human history was entering an amazing new epoch. Western civilization would become the crucible for a new era of progress. And that progress would be closely tied to the advancement of the gospel of Jesus Christ and the growth of his church. You see, God also has a strategic sense of timing.

That strategic sense of timing also applies to you and me—and our pain. At just the right time, it will be relieved. The apostle Paul went on to explain, "Because you are sons, God sent the Spirit of his Son into our hearts, the Spirit who calls out, '*Abba*, Father'" (Galatians 4:6). There is a guardian in the house. The Holy Spirit of Jesus is living in our hearts and feeling every twinge and cramp of pain. He is watching over the faith he put there. He will not let chronic pain so discourage us as to rob us of our rightful inheritance as God's heirs. Day after day he enters the fray. His Spirit joins the battle with our spirits as together we plead, "Dearest Father in heaven, grant some kind of relief." That relief may come through surgery, medication, exercise, or a raised threshold to live with pain. Or God may exercise his right to erase all our pain for all time. Relief may only come in the final victory he gives to all who remain faithful to him. It may ultimately come when we close our eyes and experience the miserable joy of a good death in Christ—a death perfectly timed to preserve a saint, because God also has a *redeeming sense of timing.*

Chapter 6

Straining Forward

Life moves in only one direction: forward. There are ups and downs and twists and turns. There is progress, and there are setbacks. But overall, everything is moving forward. The forward movement of all things is a phenomenon that God released after a thoroughly joyful existence rotted away with the last fruit on the tree of life in a cordoned-off paradise. As much as we may wish for God to take us back there, he won't. As much as we may wish he would call a halt to the direction in which things are headed, he will do it only one time, announced with the blast of a trumpet. Until then he has ordained that we must strain forward.

Forward has always been my favorite direction. I like to know which way is forward. I like to live my life headed in that direction and even get a jump on it if I can. Certainly there are great lessons to be learned from the past, or serious mistakes will be repeated. And I understand that many people are grounded in the heritage and rituals of their family or cultural legacies. Good for them! I know that straining forward produces change that can be disconcerting for some. The thought of moving forward into the unknown makes them content with the security of sitting still. But no one can really live in the past. In *The Tempest*, William Shakespeare said, "What's past is prologue." All that has gone before has merely set the stage for what is to come. Every wish that we could go back is a wasted aspiration. Each regret over past mistakes is unnecessary recrimination. We just ain't goin' back. We cannot un-ring any bells. We cannot undo any wrongs. I cannot un-lift the hay bales or big shovels of oats that weakened the lower back of my spindly adolescent frame.

And I cannot un-herniate the disc that has resulted in a life of trying to manage misery. We can only strain forward, clinging to Jesus, whose blood washed away every past mistake and whose promise to be with us to the end of the age reminds us that we are not straining forward alone. God promises to make everything new again, and the phenomenon of forwardness is getting us closer to that glorious day.

The forward movement of life was observed by Charles Darwin on the Galapagos Islands and badly misinterpreted as macroevolution. As he observed those goofy looking critters trying to adapt and struggle to survive in a hostile environment, he assumed this was a case study in the origins of life itself. He either failed, or refused, to recognize "that the whole creation has been groaning as in the pains of childbirth right up to the present time" (Romans 8:22). Rather than concocting a house-of-cards theory, Darwin and his successors should have recognized that a big delivery is still coming. And even nature is straining to be there for the blessed event. God gave all living things the capacity to strain forward. Every relentless weed in your garden is evidence of that.

Wisconsin's naturalist laureate, Aldo Leopold, saw this phenomenon in the succession of the great forests that once covered the great North. After the virgin, old growth timber was cutover for lumber or burned-over for farms, it was succeeded by different kinds of trees that sprouted from seeds that had waited patiently in the glacial soils pushed down under the floodwaters. Towering white pines gave way to scrub oaks and jack pines. Cut those over and you will see aspens, alders, ash trees, and a lot of brush volunteer. Such a progression is not the mark of evolution but a triumph of an ever-creating God, who keeps things moving forward. And always moving forward for the good of his people. So, backed up by ancient instruments, we can sing along with that last excited psalmist, "Let everything that has breath praise the LORD" (Psalm 150:6).

Life's forward movement is toward a goal. It is the goal of our salvation. It is the face-to-face reunion of the redeemed with the Redeemer. And there is only one way to pursue it. We strain forward. We strain forward in faith. The apostle Paul lived that way himself. He said, "One thing I do: Forgetting what is behind and straining toward what is ahead, I press on toward the goal to win the prize for which God has called me heavenward in Christ Jesus" (Philippians 3:13,14). The Holy Spirit caused Paul to be so absolutely sure of the outcome that his words inspire confidence in us. These excerpts from Romans chapter 8 are the manifesto of solidarity for all who are straining forward:

> The creation waits in eager expectation for the sons of God to be revealed. . . .
>
> We ourselves, who have the firstfruits of the Spirit, groan inwardly as we wait eagerly for our adoption as sons, the redemption of our bodies. For in this hope we were saved. But hope that is seen is no hope at all. Who hopes for what he already has? But if we hope for what we do not yet have, we wait for it patiently.
>
> In the same way, the Spirit helps us in our weakness. We do not know what we ought to pray for, but the Spirit himself intercedes for us with groans that words cannot express. . . .
>
> What, then, shall we say in response to this? If God is for us, who [or what] can be against us? He who did not spare his own Son, but gave him up for us all—how will he not also, along with him, graciously give us all things? . . .

> No, in all these things we are more than conquerors through him who loved us. For I am convinced that neither death nor life, neither angels nor demons, neither the present nor the future, nor any powers, [nor chronic pain], neither height nor depth, nor anything else in all creation, will be able to separate us from the love of God that is in Christ Jesus our Lord.
>
> Romans 8:19-39

Can I get an *Amen* from all who are straining forward? Can I get an *Amen* from others like me who are crippled by pain, don't know what to do or say, and can only pray, "Lord, help me. Lord, help me. Please, Lord, help me."

The ability to strain forward is a powerful gift that God gave humans. Recognizing and appreciating our amazing capacity to endure, persevere, and overcome is not capitulating to humanism. Rather, it is celebrating the human spirit as one of the jewels in the crown of God's creation. God still grants abilities to people and energizes them with fiery wills to do things that are part of his plans, great and small. The will of Luther sparked a great Reformation and put salvation by grace through faith front and center in the teaching of the church. The will of courageous immigrants tamed a new land and the will of our founding fathers constituted a great democracy.

The will of Winston Churchill held a nation together while the Nazis tried to blast it apart. Long after the Battle of Britain was over, Churchill was invited to be the graduation speaker at his alma mater. After he was introduced with accolades and a recounting of his heroic leadership, he went to the microphone. He paused and looked with steely eyes into the faces of the young graduates. Then he gave what amounted to his speech. He said in a voice roughed up by whiskey and cigars, "Never give up. Never give up. Never give up." And then he sat down. Finally, what more needed to be said? The key to success, or at least survival, is the ability to never give up. It is the ability to strain forward. That is how Churchill held his countrymen together until the Americans entered the war and turned its tide. The key was to keep straining forward.

One of the more grisly episodes in American history is the sad story of the Donner party. This group of pioneers was one of many that headed across the prairie, eager to achieve the "milk and honey" of California. Unfortunately they did everything wrong. They left at the wrong time of year. They listened to the wrong guide. Followed the wrong route. Carried along too much of the wrong stuff. Their progress stalled in the waist-deep snows of the high Sierras at what is now called Donner Pass, California. They tried everything they knew to survive. And when they could no longer strain forward together, they cannibalized one another.

Fellow pain sufferers, giving up will eat us up. And it will eat up those we love.

Since I began writing this tale, I have now had my third major back surgery. It was the only way left to strain forward. I had had several rounds of injections and ablations. None of these had provided any lasting relief. Finally, my pain doc asked what I was doing to manage the pain. I told him I was taking handfuls of over-the-counter pain relievers and lying on the couch a lot. I told him that for all these years, I had fought taking narcotic pain medication because I knew that long-term use to battle long-term pain would cause long-term problems. He called me a *narcotics virgin* and prescribed a narcotic pain reliever. The war against pain entered a new phase. It was a phase I had tried so very hard to avoid at all costs.

When I next saw my surgeon, he said, "Jason, I have only one thing left to offer you and that is to fuse the next level of your spine. It is entirely up to you."

We talked about the procedure. We talked about its potential to help and its potential to create more problems at the next level. It would require a long incision. He would remove the hardware that had been in there for 14 years. He would harvest new bone from my hip, fuse the L3-L4 level of my spine to the solid bony pile beneath it and then hold it all in place by installing some shiny new titanium rods on each side of the vertebrae.

I asked if this would be like going to the auto shop and if I would get my old parts back in a little bag. I could tell he didn't find my attempt at humor amusing.

After discussing it for a while, I told him that I thought having that surgery was inevitable. He agreed. So, we scheduled it, and all of the preparations were made. I felt joy in having another shot at relief, even though I knew the experience would be miserable. I can honestly say that I wasn't afraid of the surgery, just the outcome. That outcome remains to be seen. But I am straining forward.

Anesthesia is an amazing thing. There is no waiting while under anesthetic. The beginning and the end of surgery seem like simultaneous events. They can do things to you while you are under that you could never handle in a conscious state. And you only realize they did those things when you start coming out of it.

After seven hours of surgical procedure, a nurse's voice called to me. "Jason, you can wake up now. It's over."

That's what she thought.

Before I went under, I remember them starting a little IV on the top of my hand. When I came out of it, I had more hoses coming out of me than an old tractor's hydraulic system. I felt the breathing tube scrape across my teeth as they removed it from my throat just as I was regaining consciousness. They replaced it with a little oxygen line in my nose. There was a line going directly into the jugular vain on my neck so they could get meds into my system quickly if they had to. I had an epidural catheter implanted directly into my lumbar spine and hooked up to a morphine pump. There was another line for a blood-drain back there somewhere too. They clamped a little pulse-oxygen sensor on the end of my finger. And, as much as I hoped I would be the one surgical patient to escape it, the inevitable Foley catheter was lodged somewhere near the headwaters of my bladder.

The incision and fusion pain was excruciating. So they kept pumping morphine into my system. That made me incredibly nauseous and gave me a pounding headache. Post-surgical patients can get pretty restless. But back patients can't just toss and turn at will. I had to log-roll my entire torso very carefully with a pillow between my legs and then get boosted one way or the other by the staff. This is all very difficult to do with hoses everywhere. And wearing a hospital gown. Don't even get me started on that. They can transplant your heart, replace your hip, and remove a tumor from your brain. And this is still the best they can come up with in patient apparel? I'd rather be rolled in bubble wrap. After several days of trying to hold the back of that thing together and tug the front down every time they moved me, it finally occurred to me. The only person who hadn't seen absolutely everything was me. That was the day *my ego* grabbed hold of *my pride* and those two cowards walked out on me.

I have high respect for people employed in the medical profession. I can't say enough about the wonderful care I have received from the nurses and nursing assistants in the hospital where I was treated. I have a daughter who is a RN, and I am very proud that this is how she chose to serve the Lord with her life. It is very hard work and very important work. The nurses and nursing assistants that took care of me were generally young, professional, cheerful, respectful, and competent. Even the burly guy that gave up 20 years as a machinist to become a patient-care assistant was delightful. When he first walked in to take my vitals, he must have noticed some consternation on my face. He said, "Don't worry, they don't let me handle anything sharp."

And may God bless those zealots in the physical therapy department. It is their job to keep us straining forward. And they refuse to give up. It wasn't even 24 hours after the surgery and they were in to get me up. Were they nuts? I was ready to "code" from nausea, pain, and whole-body sweats, and they wanted to make me sit on the side of the bed and then stand up. They helped me put on my turtle-shell back brace and strapped another safety harness around my waist so they could hang on to me. I told them I wasn't sure I could do this. They got me up anyway. And then I went down . . . hard. But with their inimitable optimism, they said, "Well, that's good progress for today. We'll let you rest and come back tomorrow."

The next morning there was a rap on the door. In a pleasant singsong, they said, "Jaaa-son, it's time for ther-a-py."

I said, "I was afraid it was you guys." This time they brought a walker with them. I knew what that meant: road trip.

Soon I was moving pretty well with the walker. When I couldn't sleep at night, I got my self up and worked at putting one lead-heavy leg in front of the other to keep straining forward. Eventually they took me up to their PT gym and made me walk some more. Their primary concern was that I use proper body mechanics in every daily activity. They taught me how to get in and out of an old Dodge Neon that they had parked somehow in a fake garage on the third floor of the hospital. They showed me the proper way to get in and out of bed, to climb stairs, and climb over the tub wall to take a shower. They kept me straining forward. And because of their good work, I was able to leave the hospital within four days of major back surgery.

One night, as I was recovering at home, the phone rang next to my bed. A cheerful voice said, "Hi, Mr. Nelson. It's Greta."

I knew immediately which Greta this was. It is so cool when God brings someone special out of his clear blue at just the right time. We had moved several times since I last saw Greta and had several different phone numbers. I have no idea how she tracked me down, but I was glad she did.

She went on. "I heard you weren't doing well and just wanted you to know that it's the tenth anniversary of my transplant."

A flood of memories came back. When Greta was a high school student, she had suffered many health problems, including liver disease. She waited months for a donor. The steroids that kept her alive made her little body very puffy. She couldn't attend school regularly so we sent work and teachers to her home. One time, a clever teacher decided we should send her a video greeting from the entire school family. Every student, teacher, secretary, and custodian assembled on the bleachers of the gym. On cue we all chanted, "Greta, get betta. Greta, get betta." It was cheesy, but fun. When the transplant took place, I visited her at Children's Hospital. I have never known anyone so sick and so happy at the same time.

Her voice still rings with cheer. Greta has always been one of my heroes. Now, more than ever. She told me that since the transplant some fluky things had happened to her from all of the medications and treatments to keep her body from rejecting that liver. She developed colon cancer and serious heart trouble. But she is doing well today. And she is a teacher of two- and three-year-olds in a Lutheran early-childhood ministry. I thought to myself, who *betta* than Greta to teach little children to strain forward through all of the developmental challenges of growing up. Who better than Greta to teach little children to color within the lines and explore every corner of life within the boundaries that a loving God establishes for them? Who better than Greta to help frustrated little ones understand that life can be hard, God is love, and they just can't give up?

A great ancestor of Christ himself knew miserable joy in his life. Great David took down the giant that terrified everyone else. He enjoyed the privilege of making soothing music for his melancholy king, only to have the guy turn ornery and chuck a spear his way. He ran like a renegade and then was regaled as a hero. He buried sons because of his egregious infidelity but found great joy in the birth of another, and even greater joy in the promise of one to come much farther down his family line. He was pretty good at straining forward. But God had to establish boundaries for him so that he wouldn't strain too far. That tested his faith, gave him deep insight, and taught him to pray:

> Keep me safe, O God, for in you I take refuge. I said to the LORD, "You are my Lord; apart from you I have no good thing." . . . LORD, you have assigned me my portion and my cup; you have made my lot secure. The boundary lines have fallen for me in pleasant places; surely I have a delightful inheritance. . . . I have set the LORD always before me. Because he is at my right hand, I will not be shaken. Therefore my heart is glad and my tongue rejoices; my body also will rest secure, because you will not abandon me to the grave. . . . You have made known to me the path of life.
>
> from Psalm 16

My dear friend, when pain threatens to destroy you and you just don't know what else to do, strain forward. Just keep straining forward. Remember great David's greater Son, the Man of sorrows, who walked the way of the cross for you and me. He would have preferred to bypass that cup of suffering. But he didn't. He never faltered along the way. He kept on straining forward for us. And now he walks with us so that we can strain forward on the path of life.

Chapter 7

What Matters **Most**

On the Kenai Peninsula of Alaska there is one highway that connects the commercial center of Soldotna with the quaint fishing village of Homer. It has a very clever name: Highway 1. If one is blessed to travel it on a clear day, it is impossible to drive without humming "How Great Thou Art." Beautiful ridges covered with spruce line one side of the highway. A glimpse of a brown bear or gray wolf is possible. Eagles are everywhere. You're likely to swerve around a large, dark-eyed moose. On the other side of the highway swell the chilly, salty waters of the Cook Inlet. Beyond that rise massive volcanic cones, which are now majestic mountains like Mount Redoubt and Mount Spur. Along the way is the historic Russian settlement of Ninilchik. One of the treats of exploring Alaska is encountering this remnant of old Russian Orthodox pioneers. I guess if you live at the edge of the world, you can maintain the old ways if you want to. Their religion and culture set them apart in a state that is filled with many other groups whose cultures also set them apart. Finally, that is why many people migrate to Alaska in the first place. It is a place where there is still enough room to set yourself apart.

Ninilchik is a kind of shabby village. The streets are rutted, and the small houses provide shelter but not much else. Economic activity can be spotty in a place that may be very inhospitable. But one can't help noticing the most prominent feature of the village. On the highest hill sits a lovely little Russian Orthodox chapel. It is trimmed ornately and in good repair. It was probably one of the first things the pioneers had built and continues to be one of the things the citizens maintain the best, because it represents what has mattered most over the years to these reclusive and hardy souls.

That scene is not unique to Alaska. Settlements all over the lower 48 also feature prominent churches. These are monuments to a time when nearly every American understood what mattered most and represented it in the construction of churches. When survival is at stake, priorities are crystal clear. Calling on the name of the Lord is right near the top. That is always the mixed blessing of hard times; they make us take stock of our priorities. For many Americans their relationship with God is still what matters most. But life can get crazy. There are so many distractions and competing agendas that we easily drift into a way of living where our priorities are not real clear. And we are no longer sure of what matters most.

So, instead, we debate the issues of the moment, both those that are meaningful and those that are truly insignificant. Christian liberty and American freedom permit us to have those debates. This is a precious right. The ability to conduct them with vigor and civility should be practiced. How do we best respond to the threat of terror? What is the future of Social Security? Which are better, Fords or Chevys? Does it taste great, or is it less filling? Should we consume fewer carbs or eat less fat?

Even in the church it can sometimes be hard to differentiate what matters most. Many tense debates have faded with the memories of aging members. Should we use the common cup or individual glasses? Will we have a potluck or hire a caterer? Do we build a new church or wait our turn to be carried out of the old one? Do we adopt a new hymnal or sing the old songs we grew up with?

Let us have our debates with respect for one another and without name-calling. Our convictions are important. We are right to exercise the courage of our convictions. God uses human conviction. Very often it accomplishes his purposes. But we must also be aware that our convictions can deceive us. They can take us to extreme places if we are not careful. Then constructive debates become destructive controversies. So often those controversies are unnecessary. They are skirmishes among people at the far edges of what matters most. Wise people eventually ask, How much does this really matter? We should listen to them more often. And where it applies unquestionably, let us settle the matter with final submission to the authority of God's Holy Word. Let us recommit ourselves to what matters most.

That is where pain can be a great simplifier. Pain quickly focuses us on what matters most. When we have felt enough pain, we are ready to change what we were not ready to change before. When the pain of addiction is just so much worse than the pain of sobriety, the addict is ready to change. When the risks of maintaining the status quo overshadow the pain of charting a new direction, the organization is ready to change. Some individuals or groups aren't ready to change because they haven't felt enough pain yet. When we have felt enough pain, we think about some things so much more and other things so much less. When we have felt enough pain, we are better able to clean out the attics of our existence and treasure what is essential. By the time pain has its way with us, there is only energy to care about what matters most. I can't help thinking that the long-running dispute in the Middle East over the West Bank could be resolved if every Palestinian and every Israeli had a lumbar fusion.

There was a time when I had passion for a lot of things. I didn't always prioritize them carefully and pursued them all aggressively. But that is not the case right now. At the end of the day there is just enough energy for the miserable joy of appreciating what matters most and only what matters most. The constant love and support of such a good wife, the achievements and self-sufficiency of wonderful children with whom God has blessed me richly, the genuine concern of true friends, the good vibe of a sunny day, and the salvation of souls that are so precious to our God.

The salvation of souls is what matters most.

When God asked his triune self, What am I willing to die for? There was only one answer. It was people. God was willing to die for people. He was willing to die for people who can be stinky and disgusting and rebellious by nature. God wants nothing more than to bring people to himself. That is why Jesus shed his blood. It was real lifeblood that had a type and hemoglobin count. It was the blood of a dying man and the living God, hemorrhaging down a horrible cross. It was blood that proved the paternity of God for all mankind—his DNA *is* love. That is what saving people meant to God. He would not have paid that price for any other reason, because there is no ambiguity for God about what matters most. Nothing matters more than the salvation of your soul and my soul. Nothing matters more than the salvation of the souls of people who don't even know their souls need saving.

I wonder if the thorn in Paul's flesh helped the apostle understand what mattered most. He sure taught the most important things in life clearly. It had to be an overwhelming task for this relatively new convert to plant the churches of infant Christianity across the then-known world. Those churches existed within complex cultures, steeped in a profusion of beliefs and syncretistic practices, many of which put the gospel at risk. No sooner would Paul leave a new church behind than he would learn that they were falling back into deadly, old patterns. Paul would teach his heart out only to have some of the very Christians he taught sell out to their own sinful longings. But the Spirit of God was with Paul. And that Holy Spirit inspired Paul with words to help people grow in faith and understand what matters most.

The Galatians were a case in point. After Paul left them, some manipulating *Judaizers* came in. Their message was a mishmash of co-opting the gospel with old Jewish law. Their message left people less than totally dependent on Christ. They said, You may belong to Christ, but you are still obligated to the old ways and the old laws of our Jewish tradition; and the line for circumcisions forms right here.

Paul was heartbroken to learn that many of those beloved Galatian converts got in line. They were willing to swap their fresh, new freedom in Christ for an all-too-human slavishness to works and rituals. Paul didn't mince words. In a take-no-prisoners discourse, Paul drove a stake in the ground for Christian liberty, and he clarified people's confusion about what matters most. "The only thing that counts," Paul wrote, "is faith expressing itself through love" (Galatians 5:6).

In a life where lots of things can matter, there is only one thing that counts. That is faith. The only thing that counts is the belief in your heart that what you know in your head is the absolute truth. Jesus is the Savior of your soul and the piloting Lord of your life. Since that is the only thing that counts, God didn't entrust bestowing it to anyone other than himself. It was his Spirit's work through his Word, and in Baptism, that created in you the ability to trust the Lord with all your heart. He took the initiative and reached out with gentle fingers and touched that hidden place where you believe. And you believed. Then he willed for your believing to grow. He intervenes in your life with things like pain to make sure it does.

Pain causes us to dive deeply into God's Word to learn more of what it teaches. That Word is the means God uses to build us up and believe even more so that we can cope even better. We need to really understand what counts when our pain is at its worst.

Taking Holy Communion often allows us to taste and see that the Lord is good, even when pain and medicine leave a very bitter taste in our mouths. The bread and wine and body and blood of our once-sacrificed Lord are sacred reminders that Jesus suffered a grim death for us and continues to strengthen our dependence on him and our bond with one another. Believe me. I know the confusion pain causes and how it diffuses clear thinking. But the only thing that counts is faith. And we need to take advantage of every opportunity to keep it strong.

And, at the very same time, the only thing that counts is faith expressing itself. God did not give us faith so that it could be a private matter. Nor is it a festival thing to be brought out just on special occasions. As the Holy Spirit works, our confidence in Christ builds up big on the inside. Bigger even than our pain. And then it starts pressuring for release. And frequently that need to give expression to our faith—that building pressure—occurs in the simple things of day-to-day living. My point is that living in pain is not a pass on living for Christ. It just makes living for him a more strenuous exercise of one's faith.

When you and everyone around you can see things aren't going well, that is the perfect time for faith to express itself.

Faith expresses itself in praises and not cursing. Faith expresses itself in kindness and not complaint. Faith expresses itself in self-sacrifice and not self-pity. Faith expresses itself in hope and not despair. And faith expresses itself in sincere invitations for others to learn what you have learned and to believe what you believe. Let a world that sees you in pain also see in you the only thing that counts.

And the only thing that counts is faith, expressing itself, . . . *in love.* God has established one criterion for the way in which faith should be expressed. That is in love. Dear friend, there is no uncertainty here either: *Love always feels like love.* For the person expressing it and for the person receiving it, love always feels like love.

Oh, it is true that expressions of love can vary. Love can be tender or it can be tough. Love can be permissive or it can be firm. Love can be shouted from the rooftops or whispered in an ear. Love can prompt expensive gifts or be expressed in simple things. But upon the further review of mental and emotional replay, love will always feel like love. A strict parent can genuinely say I sent you to your room because I love you. And after sputtering to himself for a while, a child who has cooled down will know the loving motive was real. Love always feels like love.

If words or actions haunt you because there was a love claim, but it just doesn't feel like love; it wasn't love. It is a contemptible fraud to do harm and call it love. Physical abuse is never love. Sexual abuse is never love. Mean-spirited exclusion is never love. Selfish demands are never love. Manipulation is never love. On either end they never feel like love. To say otherwise is a damnable lie. Faith expresses itself in love. The apostle John did not leave any loophole in this discussion. "Whoever does not love does not know God, because God is love" (1 John 4:8).

Why such strong words? Our pain can hurt others. Pain people must be on guard. Pain can make people mean. It can make people self-centered. It can cause people to focus only on themselves or on no one at all. It can convince them they have a right to do or say something selfish or something hurtful. Pain can make it very difficult to express faith in love.

To see faith expressed in love, we read on with John to discover the real essence of love. "This is how God showed his love among us: He sent his one and only Son into the world that we might live through him. This is love: not that we loved God, but that he loved us and sent his Son as an atoning sacrifice for our sins. Dear friends, since God so loved us, we also ought to love one another" (1 John 4:9-11).

The atoning sacrifice of Christ is the absolute standard for love. To bind faith with love one must take up the cross of Christ. That cross is what reconciles us to God and with one another when we fail to express our faith in loving actions and words. In Jesus' cross we find forgiveness from

God and for one another. God may not remove our pain until we meet him face-to-face. But he has already removed the shame and guilt of failing to express our faith in love. And his love for us empowers us to order our lives around the only thing that counts. Do not underestimate the soothing effect on pain when faith expresses itself in love.

In the college I attended, every education student was required to take piano and organ lessons. This expectation came out of the noble ideal that all good Christian teachers should be able to play the piano and organ. Lack of aptitude really didn't matter. The dear lady who drew the short straw that made me her student was dying of cancer. My progress at the keyboard was so slow it hardly existed. Each succeeding lesson became a rehash of the previous lesson. How hard she tried to get two awkward hands and two clumsy feet to work together to play the same song! A lesser woman would have grabbed me by the throat and said, "Listen, you putz, I don't have much time left, and I am wasting far too much of it on you." But she didn't. She was patient. She was persistent. She was kind. And she kept teaching me like it mattered.

When she went to the hospital to die, it was widely reported that she visited other patients and tried to encourage them with the only thing that counts—faith expressing itself in love. In her final hours, her primary concern was for the welfare of others. I cannot remember one thing she taught me about playing the organ, but I will never ever forget the lesson she taught me about what matters most.

Chapter 8

A Survival Guide for "Pain People"

Pray without ceasing

We have all watched this scene in a movie: Family and friends are huddled around the sickbed of a loved one. The doctor says with gravity, "We have done everything we can. All we can do now is pray." Why is it that even Christian people view prayer as the last resort? If all else fails, pray. I have fallen into that trap. Actually prayer is appropriate at both the beginning and the end of a survivor's experience with pain.

God promises that prayer changes things. I have been very grateful for the many friends and relatives who have been praying for me. And I am grateful that their prayers have been bolder than mine. They are asking God to take my pain away completely. I have been timid. I have sheepishly asked God for just a little relief. Maybe I haven't gotten much relief because I haven't expected much. God invites us to come to him boldly and confidently as children come to a loving father. Let's recommit ourselves to praying like we mean it.

Keep moving

Much of the pain sensation involves muscles. Nerves send messages to the brain. The brain sorts them out and sends messages to muscles, and then something happens. In many pain syndromes, muscles spasm, ache, cramp, or feel weak. That experience causes us not to want to move much at all. It hurts when we move. Now, if moving can do more damage to a joint or injury, then we must be very careful. But with chronic pain syndromes, movement is important. It can strengthen muscles that support the joints, reducing the irritation of nerves that send the pain signals to the brain. The right kind of movement can help ease pain.

Make the best use of the best time

Most pain sufferers know that pain ebbs and flows. There are good days and bad days. In some cases there are bad days and worse days. There are times of the day when pain is in the background and times of the day when it is front and center. Pain does not mean we cannot be productive. It just means we have to make the most productive use of the times when our pain is less. If we are blessed with a decent night's sleep, the first thing in the morning may be a good time. Over the years that I have been battling pain, that has proven to be my most productive time. For instance, if I am going to do any writing, I have to do a little when I first get up. My capacity to sit is very limited. So, I sit a little the first thing in the morning. I know from experience that later I will need to try to keep moving or lie down.

Be your own advocate

As Christians, we value selflessness and humility. We are not comfortable with making us our own cause. But we must face a hard reality when dealing with employers, or medical institutions, insurance agencies, government, or other bureaucracies. We cannot assume people are going to do what they say they will do. We cannot assume people are doing what they are supposed to do. Even if they've told you they will do it. I don't want to be cynical, but there is only one person you can ultimately trust to connect all of the dots. That is you. We pain people will often need to shoulder the responsibility of being our own advocates and follow up with the details.

I learned this the hard way in applying for disability benefits. A decision was slow in coming. So I checked on things. I discovered that the hospital would not send necessary records to the insurance company because the insurance company wasn't using the correct request form to comply with new privacy regulations. They didn't tell this to anyone; they just didn't send the records. I suspected that the decision regarding benefits was overdue. When I did decide to check on things, the insurance company told me they weren't getting the records they needed from the doctors and hospital. The hospital told me I would have to contact the service they hired to handle medical records. Those people told me to tell the insurance company to get its act together and use the right forms. I pleaded with people on the phone to do what they needed to do for my sake. Finally, I went to the records department, picked them up, and mailed them myself. It was frustrating and time consuming, but the people who would have suffered if that decision would have been allowed to linger any longer would have been my family.

Here is the lesson I learned from this experience: *Even though you have filled out all the forms and met all the deadlines, don't assume no news is good news. Regularly, persistently, and politely double-check on things.* I have made it a habit to make follow-up phone calls to confirm all materials have been received and to inquire if anything else needs to be done.

Work with your doctors

There was a time when the relationship of patients with doctors was passive. Doctors were one of the priestly classes who knew secrets common folks didn't know. But the patient-centered approach to medicine and the information age have made the doctor-patient relationship a partnership. As much as we depend on our doctors, our doctors also depend on us to give them the right information and accurate feedback on treatments. Working with doctors is work. And we must learn our role as patients.

Part of the work is learning new things and gathering information. The Internet is a tremendous blessing in this area. Over the past two years I was introduced to new medications and new terminology. When one of my pain specialists began talking about radio frequency nerve ablation, I needed to know everything I could. At first I didn't even know how to spell it. So my first searches were fruitless. Eventually I connected. I read reports on the procedure itself and postings from people who had experienced it. Many of those postings were encouraging. When I had the first ablation, I made a point to review with the doctor my understanding of how it worked. I asked, "Do I have this right? You are going to insert a probe up against my vertebrae where the sensory nerve is located. You will be doing this under live X ray. You won't be able to see the nerve, but you will see bony structures that will give you an idea where the nerve is supposed to be. Then you will turn up the juice and coagulate the nerve, disconnecting it from the facet joint. When the nerve is ablated, it won't be able to send the pain signal to the brain, and eventually the brain will stop sending the pain signal along nerve pathways in other places."

He said, "Exactly." I was pleased with myself because I had rendered this speech under mild sedation. I knew what to say, even under sedation, because I had read about it on the Internet. Two sites that proved very valuable for me were SpineUniverse.com and WebMD.com.

I worked closely with my surgeon until I could assess my own situation. He is not the kind of person to push things on his patients. He is more inclined to gently lead them to understand their own situation, and then he confirms their understanding. I had my third back surgery only after he agreed that I had a good understanding of my condition.

Many pain sufferers will jump from doctor to doctor looking for help that has been hard to find. We can easily believe we are not getting relief because we are not seeing the right doctor. It is true that not all doctors have the same level of knowledge and skill. A second opinion or new doctor may be necessary. But understand your condition first.

It's true, the back is very complex, and back problems are hard to diagnose. The results of surgery are often less than perfect. Over the years I have seen several doctors. My family doctor referred me to a pain specialist and an orthopedic surgeon. The pain specialist worked with me for several months, and the orthopedic surgeon consulted with me. When I began to suspect another surgery might become necessary, I returned to the neurology surgeon who had operated on me twice before. I have great confidence in him. I stayed with him over the long term as he ordered scans, referred me to another pain specialist, and directed my treatment. If you have confidence in your doctors, stay with them. They know your history. You may get quicker relief than you would if you were to start all over with different doctors. The practice of medicine involves a process of elimination. It may not make sense to start that process over from the beginning with someone new.

Don't be afraid to ask questions and offer your opinion of your situation and treatment options. Most doctors will listen. Stay focused on your primary ailment. When we are hurting it is easy to get sidetracked and believe everything is falling apart. Usually it isn't. Write things down so you'll remember. Keep a journal of your pain so that you can describe what makes it worse and what makes it better. Listen to your own body.

My pain specialist was using injections to try to provide some relief and as a way of diagnosing the origin of my pain. Among these were caudal space (tailbone) injections. Because I had so much low pain and trouble sitting, he thought this was worth trying. He did one and there was no change. He wanted to try another injection at the next appointment. But I also felt so much discomfort in the joint above the fusion. Previous facet joint injections and the nerve ablation at that level provided some temporary relief. I politely asked him if he could try an epidural space injection at that level instead of the caudal space injection he planned to do.

He said, "It's your back, and I will try anything that might help you."

That injection hit pay dirt for about three days. And it gave even stronger evidence that a strong source of my pain was the L3-L4 level of my spine.

I pray for my doctors. I ask God to guide their minds, their hearts, and their hands. Obviously, I need them to make the right decisions on my behalf. I want God to guide them. I want God looking over their shoulders.

I also send my doctors and their staff thank-you notes. I am truly grateful for their efforts in my behalf, and I want them to know that. My surgeon and I have also talked about Jesus.

In a conversation that he started about Mel Gibson's movie *The Passion of the Christ*, he said, "The most important thing is that he rose again."

Part of my confidence in him is that he has confidence in Christ. My thank-you note to him featured the words of Hebrews 6:10: "He will not forget your work and the love you have shown him as you have helped his people and continue to help them." At the next visit, I saw that note taped inside my file.

What about the pills?

I have great anxiety over using narcotic medications to battle pain. I knew early on that I would be fighting pain for years, maybe even a lifetime. I did not want to be in line with Brett Favre, Rush Limbaugh, or Matthew Perry going into drug rehab because of addiction to narcotic painkillers. But I also know a person just needs a break from pain. It is just impossible to gut it out all the time.

My first pain doc prescribed an antiseizure medication. The strategy was to ramp up the dosage until I felt little pain. By the time I got to 3,600 milligrams per day, I wasn't feeling much of anything. It did enable me to function for one year in my final position in church work. But I was mentally dull and had absolutely no energy left at the end of the day.

Prior to my last surgery, my second pain doc gave me one of the newer narcotic pain medications. It was a combination of an opium derivative and acetaminophen. It helped me get some things done before I went in for surgery, but there were side effects. The maximum dosage was eight per day. I never took more than three per day. If I took three per day for two days in a row I was nauseous and had a splitting headache. My body does not tolerate any of the morphine derivatives well. Yet I know some pain people must wear a morphine pump just to have any quality of life. The reality is that pain people have to make some hard choices. Sometimes those choices will boil down to which form of suffering is preferable on any given day.

Adapt when you can

Pain people may have to adapt their lifestyles or use adaptive devices just to function. If a cane takes some stress off hurting joints, use it. If a walker helps, use that. I worked for two years standing up because I couldn't sit. Then when I could no longer stand, I had to give up working. That was a heartbreaking way to adapt.

As I recover from my third surgery, I have to wear a rigid brace for three to six months until the bone graft heals. And then after that I still won't be able to bend at the waist. So, I got a grabber. It's a long tube with two fingers on one end and a pistol grip with a trigger on the other. When I squeeze the trigger, the fingers come together. If I drop something, I use the grabber to pick it up. And I drop a lot of things. I can easily pick things off the floor like my shoes, socks, and most of my lunch.

Do something you like

I have a friend who says, "You can get through anything if you have something to look forward to." There is so much truth in that statement. That is why the morale of the American worker changes so noticeably from Monday to Friday. Most people have something to look forward to on the weekend. We cope with difficulty better when we have something to look forward to than when we don't.

The pain experience changes what we look forward to. Maybe it will be a little thing like sitting in a hot tub. That is important because the pleasure and relaxation change the pain experience and remind us it is still possible to have some pleasant moments. Maybe we have big things to look forward to, like attending the graduations of children or one of their sporting events. Or maybe it will be some favorite thing to look forward to like going out to eat. While pain may still be a constant companion, it will be easier to ignore it for a while if we are doing something we enjoy doing.

Of course, we all have something really big to look forward to. Because of Jesus, we look forward to heaven.

You can get through anything if you have something to look forward to in faith. All problems are temporary. All pain has an end in sight. In a worst-case scenario, some pain can last a lifetime. But Paul put even such extreme forms of pain into perspective when he wrote, "I consider that our present sufferings are not worth comparing with the glory that will be revealed in us" (Romans 8:18). And remember, Paul could say that having had a lifetime of experience with pain.

Help someone else

One of the most fulfilling things anyone can do is to help other people find fulfillment. Pain may restrict our ability to serve, but it does not necessarily eliminate our ability to serve. Being a *living sacrifice* is our spiritual act of worship. A big part of showing our love and reverence for God is carried out in real life in the way we help other people. Serving others is a sacrifice we make willingly. Pain people may feel the stinging burden of that sacrifice more than others, but there is nothing that takes our minds off of our problems better than devoting ourselves to helping others with theirs. It may take some of us more time and experimentation to know how we will be able to serve. Saying a prayer, sending a card, making a meal, calling on people, maybe even writing a book could be among the offerings we make as living sacrifices.

Chapter 9

The **Flight** of Healing

It is a miracle. Under normal, predictable circumstances, the body, mind, and spirit can hold itself together for 80 years, give or take. Over a lifetime the miraculous power of healing allows skin to grow together, bones to mend, lungs to clear, infections to disappear, and inflammations to settle down. In our larger being, we can get over breaking up with a girlfriend or boyfriend and even get through the loss of a spouse. We can recover from a personal breakdown and overcome the break up of a family. No matter what is bruised, broken, or shattered in our lives, there is healing.

I think healing is a residue of Eden. The first bodies God formed out of the dust and breathed life into were designed to last forever. The descendents of Adam lived several hundred years before the most severe consequence of sin eventually overtook the regenerative force God had created in people. During especially hard times in history, life expectancy was fairly short. In especially inhospitable terrains, it still is. But all indications are that we are bouncing back. We are benefiting from cleaner air and water, more nutritious food, and healthier living. Our children will very likely live longer than we will. And many of us will outlive the ability of parts of our body to hang in there with us. Today we can get knees, hips, and other things replaced. It is a miracle that even though we are ultimately headed back to the dust from which we came, we are now living longer and there is so much more healing that goes on along the way.

But healing takes time. Especially when the nerves are involved. And given the amazing tangle of nerves that run electrical service from the brain to all parts of the body, the nerves are almost always involved. From the hypersensitive little receptors in our fingertips to the heavy sciatic nerve coming out of our lumbar spine, nerves are involved in injury, and they are involved in healing. That is often why healing takes time.

My surgeon is an expert with nerves and has described them for me a number of ways. Once he told me they had a consistency like toothpaste. We can imagine squeezing a line of toothpaste on the counter. Very slowly and carefully it could be lifted with delicate instruments and moved. Very easily it could be damaged in the process. A dent in a line of toothpaste is going to be there for a while. Probably a very long while before an invisible change in surface tensions would allow it to regain its normal form.

Another time he told me that nerves are like elephants. They never forget. As a result they send pain signals even after the problem is resolved. And because nerves don't forget, neither do we. We feel pain long after we should. And that becomes yet another aspect of recovery.

Somewhere in the mix of wounds, nerves, and memories is the emotional side of healing. As much as anything, it is that side of healing that takes time. And, it is that side of healing that creates the opportunity for joy to overcome misery.

It is now nearly two years since my last back surgery. I am happy to report there has been some healing. At least that is how I feel most days. It seems that I can sit a little longer, stand a little more comfortably, and sleep a little better than I did a year ago. I am praying that next year at this time I will be able to say the same thing. I have been through this before, and I know that this kind of healing takes time. I know that it takes time for muscles that have been severed and spread to knit back together. It takes time for tissue that has been peeled away from bone to reattach. It takes time for nerves to forget. I also know that the measure of healing will be scaled to my ability to function, and not to how much pain I feel. How we function is a better measure for healing than how we feel. In the end, it may be the only measure that matters because it is double edged. It cuts both ways. Am I smiling because I am happy, or am I happy because I am smiling? Am I functioning better because I am feeling less pain, or am I feeling less pain because I am functioning better? The answer to both is yes.

Sometimes Jesus went with that measure of healing. His primary concern was always for spiritual and eternal things. He also pushed people to get on with their lives because he knew the two were woven together. When the devoted companions of the paralytic of Capernaum lowered their crippled friend through the roof, Jesus saw faith and forgave sin. That took care of this poor man's ultimate need. Being right with God is just more important than being able to walk. Then Jesus went on to deal with the suspicious and critical thoughts of the onlookers. Eventually he turned his attention back to the man who was healed. Jesus didn't spend much time processing what occurred with him. He didn't refer him for rabbinical counseling so the man could come to grips with this wonderfully traumatic change in his life. He made no mention of vocational rehabilitation. He simply told the man to get up and go home. In full view of everyone, the man did. He began to function immediately.

My father suffered from a different kind of chronic pain. It was the pain of mental and emotional illness. It was the pain of total nervous breakdowns and all of the memory tremors that followed seismic life wounds. It is hard to know whether a very difficult childhood caused these problems or if these problems caused a very difficult childhood. The details are a story of their own. But his entire adult life was a grueling ground war to gain enough healing to function. There were always setbacks that frightened him and the rest of us. We all understood the consequences of losing the battle. We saw him in such pain of mind and spirit that he couldn't function. But by the end of his life, there had been enough healing. Not total healing, but enough healing. He stayed at jobs for longer periods of time. He was less volatile in temperament. His love for his family was unambiguous. His faith in Jesus now allows him to rest in peace. But each and every day of his life was a struggle for that healing. And it took a lifetime for it to occur.

In addition to requiring a lot of time, healing can also be such a flighty thing. Its trajectory is less like a rocket's and more like a butterfly's. There are certainly some things that heal in a straight line. The X rays show that my new bone fusion at L3-L4 is just about healed. Right on schedule. But the discomfort it is supposed to alleviate comes and goes. There is progress, and there are setbacks. There are better days, and there are worse days. And there is a symbiotic mind-body relationship. When I think I am making progress, I feel better physically and emotionally. And when I think I might be deteriorating one more time, the anxiety produces frightening sensations in every corner of my being. This is the fragile and irregular flight of healing that is the end game for so much of what hurts so many of us.

The flight of healing may be unpredictable, but the source of healing is sure. It is a loving God who moves us from heartache to healing. He hovered over the primordial mass and healed its chaos with an orderly creation. He hovered over the damning rift between humanity and himself and healed it by sacrificing his only Son. He hovers over the church and heals error in Christian teaching with reformation. He hovers over the nations and heals the destruction of wars with new chapters in history. God hovers over our homes and heals our broken relationships. God hovers over our hospital beds and heals our diseases. He and his angels hover over everything. He hovers with mercy, truth, power, and justice. He hovers over wastelands of misery and transforms them with seeds of joy. There is healing in his wings.

A Final **Blessing**

May the Great Physician and Savior of
your soul be kind with your body.
Don't let pain cause despair; make it the
proving ground of faith.
Have a good cry when you need one and
a good laugh when you need one.
May you find a comfortable way to get
through each day
And a comfortable position to help you
sleep through the night.
See time as an ally that makes healing
more likely.
Use God's Word to drive off Satan when he
tries to make mischief through your pain.
Pray continually, hope fervently, and never
give up.
Don't let pain alter your personality;
instead, let it develop your character.
Find an outlet for every good desire and
a good design for every dream.
Replace doubt with trust and loneliness
with friendship.
Reach out to others and reach back
when others reach out to you.
Feel alive and well when a loved
one touches you tenderly.
Accept that miserable joy is better
than no joy at all.
Believe with all your heart that these
days of miserable joy are short
And that soon they will be replaced with
perfect joy that never ends,
When you will see God face-to-face.

CPSIA information can be obtained at www.ICGtesting.com
Printed in the USA
LVOW04s0627190914

404878LV00002B/5/P

9 780810 017498